COPING WITH ADHD:

A GUIDE FOR PARENTS AND CAREGIVERS

DR. MELISSA P. NELSON

TABLE OF CONTENTS

Preface

Dear Parents and Caregivers,

Welcome to "Coping with ADHD: A Guide for Parents and Caregivers." This guide has been created with the understanding that raising a child with Attention-Deficit/Hyperactivity Disorder (ADHD) can present unique challenges and complexities. We aim to provide you with valuable insights, practical strategies, and support to help you navigate the journey of supporting your child with ADHD.

Parenting or caregiving for a child with ADHD can be both rewarding and demanding. You may have witnessed your child's unique strengths, creativity, and enthusiasm, while also facing the struggles that come with attention difficulties, impulsivity, and hyperactivity. It is essential to remember that you are not alone on this journey. Many other parents and caregivers share similar experiences, and professionals are available to provide guidance and support.

This guide is designed to offer you a comprehensive understanding of ADHD and equip you with strategies to manage its various aspects. From understanding the basics of

ADHD to recognizing symptoms, seeking a diagnosis, and exploring treatment options, we will provide you with a solid foundation of knowledge. We will address common challenges related to ADHD, such as managing behavior, supporting academic progress, and promoting social skills. Additionally, we will touch on coexisting conditions, transitions to adolescence and adulthood, and the importance of taking care of yourself as a parent or caregiver.

Throughout this guide, we encourage you to approach each topic with an open mind and a willingness to adapt the strategies to suit your unique circumstances. Remember that every child with ADHD is an individual with their own strengths, needs, and preferences. The strategies discussed in this guide are not one-size-fits-all solutions, but rather starting points that can be tailored to your child's specific requirements.

As you embark on this journey, it is important to remember that you are doing an incredible job. Parenting or caregiving for a child with ADHD requires patience, empathy, and resilience. Celebrate your successes, no matter how small, and acknowledge the progress you and your child make together.

Above all, keep in mind that this guide is meant to serve as a resource and a support system for you. Trust your instincts, seek professional guidance when needed, and remember that you are your child's greatest advocate.

Thank you for your commitment and dedication to supporting your child with ADHD. Together, we can create an environment where they can thrive and reach their full potential.

Chapter 1: Introduction to ADHD: Understanding the Basics

Attention-Deficit/Hyperactivity Disorder (ADHD) is a neurodevelopmental disorder that affects individuals across various age groups. It is characterized by persistent patterns of inattention, hyperactivity, and impulsivity, which can significantly impact daily functioning and quality of life. This introductory guide aims to provide a better understanding of ADHD by exploring its definition, symptoms, prevalence, diagnosis, as well as dispelling common myths and misconceptions surrounding the disorder.

Defining ADHD and its Symptoms:
ADHD is a complex condition that involves difficulties with attention, impulse control, and hyperactivity. Individuals with ADHD often struggle to sustain attention, easily become distracted, and may exhibit a tendency to switch between tasks frequently. They may also struggle with organizing and completing tasks, forgetfulness, and difficulty following instructions. Hyperactivity in ADHD manifests as excessive restlessness, fidgeting, and an inability to stay seated or engage in quiet activities. Impulsivity can

lead to impulsive decision-making, interrupting others, and difficulty waiting for turns. These symptoms vary in intensity and presentation among individuals, and can manifest differently in children, adolescents, and adults.

Prevalence and Diagnosis:

ADHD is a common neurodevelopmental disorder, affecting people worldwide. According to the Diagnostic and Statistical Manual of Mental Disorders (DSM-5), the prevalence of ADHD is estimated to be around 5-10% in children and 2-5% in adults. However, it is important to note that these numbers may vary across different populations and diagnostic criteria.

Diagnosing ADHD involves a comprehensive evaluation conducted by a qualified healthcare professional, such as a psychiatrist or psychologist. The diagnostic process typically includes gathering information from various sources, such as the individual, parents or caregivers (in the case of children), teachers, and other relevant individuals. The symptoms must be present in multiple settings and significantly impact the individual's functioning to receive a diagnosis. A thorough assessment helps rule out other possible explanations for the observed symptoms, such as medical conditions, learning disabilities, or psychological disorders.

Myths and Misconceptions about ADHD:
ADHD has been subject to several myths and misconceptions that can contribute to misunderstandings and stigma. One common myth is that ADHD is merely a result of laziness or a lack of discipline. In reality, ADHD is a neurobiological condition influenced by a combination of genetic, environmental, and neurological factors.

Another misconception is that ADHD only affects children, and individuals outgrow it as they reach adulthood. However, ADHD often persists into adulthood, although symptoms may evolve and manifest differently. Many adults with ADHD continue to face challenges in areas such as time management, organization, and impulsivity.

Additionally, the belief that ADHD is overdiagnosed or used as an excuse for poor behavior is a myth. While accurate diagnosis is essential, studies suggest that ADHD is still underdiagnosed and undertreated in many cases.

By dispelling these myths and misconceptions, it becomes easier to foster a more accurate understanding of ADHD and provide support and resources to those who may be affected by the condition.

In conclusion, ADHD is a neurodevelopmental disorder characterized by inattention, hyperactivity, and impulsivity. It affects individuals across various age groups and can significantly impact daily functioning. Understanding the symptoms, prevalence, and diagnostic process helps break down misconceptions and fosters a more supportive environment for individuals with ADHD.

Chapter 2: Recognizing ADHD in Children: Signs and Symptoms

Identifying Attention-Deficit/Hyperactivity Disorder (ADHD) in children is crucial for early intervention and support. Recognizing the signs and symptoms can help parents, caregivers, and educators understand the challenges faced by children with ADHD. This section will outline the common behavioral and cognitive symptoms of ADHD, discuss the differences in symptoms between boys and girls, and highlight the co-occurring conditions often associated with ADHD.

Common Behavioral and Cognitive Symptoms:
Children with ADHD typically exhibit a range of behavioral and cognitive symptoms that can significantly impact their daily lives.
These symptoms fall into three main categories: **inattention**, **hyperactivity**, and **impulsivity**.

1. Inattention:
  - Difficulty sustaining attention on tasks or activities, easily distracted
  - Trouble organizing tasks and belongings

- Forgetfulness and frequently losing necessary items
- Avoidance or dislike of tasks requiring sustained mental effort
- Tendency to become overwhelmed or disengaged when faced with complex or lengthy tasks

2. Hyperactivity:

- Restlessness and constant fidgeting
- Inability to remain seated or stay in one place for long
- Excessive talking and difficulty engaging in quiet activities
- Difficulty waiting for turns and interrupting others
- Impulsive behavior without considering potential consequences

3. Impulsivity:

- Acting without thinking, leading to accidents or injuries
- Difficulty waiting for their turn in games or activities
- Interrupting or intruding on conversations and activities of others
- Impatience and difficulty with delayed gratification

Differences in Symptoms between Boys and Girls:
ADHD symptoms can vary between boys and girls, leading to potential differences in how the disorder presents itself. Boys often display more hyperactive and impulsive

behaviors, drawing attention to their difficulties. On the other hand, girls may exhibit more internalizing symptoms and present as daydreamers or socially withdrawn, leading to their symptoms being overlooked or attributed to other causes. Girls with ADHD may also have higher rates of co-occurring conditions, such as anxiety or depression.

Co-occurring Conditions:
Children with ADHD frequently experience co-occurring conditions that can further complicate their lives.
Some of the commonly observed conditions include:

1. Anxiety and Depression: Children with ADHD may experience heightened levels of anxiety and depression due to their challenges with attention, impulsivity, and social interactions.

2. Learning Disabilities: ADHD can often coexist with learning disabilities, making it more difficult for children to succeed academically. Difficulties with reading, writing, and math may be present.

3. Oppositional Defiant Disorder (ODD) and Conduct Disorder (CD): ODD and CD are behavioral disorders that can occur alongside ADHD. Children with ODD may exhibit defiance, hostility, and refusal to comply with rules and authority figures. CD involves more serious behaviors such as aggression, lying, and a disregard for others' rights.

4. Autism Spectrum Disorder (ASD): Some children with ADHD may also have ASD, characterized by challenges in social communication and interaction, as well as restricted and repetitive behaviors.

Recognizing these co-occurring conditions is crucial in providing comprehensive support and appropriate interventions for children with ADHD.

In conclusion, recognizing ADHD in children involves identifying common behavioral and cognitive symptoms, understanding potential differences in symptoms between boys and girls, and recognizing the co-occurring conditions that often accompany ADHD. By being aware of these signs and symptoms, parents, caregivers, and educators can take appropriate steps to provide the necessary support and interventions to help children with ADHD thrive.)

Chapter 3: Getting an ADHD Diagnosis: The Evaluation Process

Receiving a proper ADHD diagnosis is essential for understanding and addressing the challenges faced by individuals with Attention-Deficit/Hyperactivity Disorder (ADHD). The evaluation process involves professional assessments and working closely with healthcare professionals and specialists.

This section will discuss the importance of a professional assessment, the types of assessments and evaluations used, and the collaborative approach to working with healthcare professionals.

Importance of Professional Assessment:

A professional assessment is crucial for an accurate ADHD diagnosis. While self-assessment tools and online questionnaires can provide some initial insights, only a qualified healthcare professional, such as a psychiatrist, psychologist, or pediatrician, can conduct a comprehensive evaluation. They have the expertise to differentiate ADHD symptoms from other conditions with similar features and determine the most appropriate course of treatment.

Types of Assessments and Evaluations:

The evaluation process for ADHD typically involves various assessments and evaluations, which may include:

1. Clinical Interviews: Healthcare professionals conduct interviews with the individual seeking diagnosis, as well as parents or caregivers (in the case of children), to gather information about the individual's history, symptoms, and functioning in different settings.

2. Rating Scales and Questionnaires: Standardized rating scales, such as the ADHD Rating Scale, are used to assess the presence and severity of ADHD symptoms. These questionnaires are typically completed by parents, teachers, and the individual themselves, providing a comprehensive view of symptoms across various settings.

3. Medical and Developmental History: Reviewing the individual's medical history, including any previous diagnoses or treatments, as well as developmental milestones, can provide important insights into the onset and progression of symptoms.

4. Behavioral Observations: Observing the individual's behavior in different settings, such as school or home, can help identify ADHD-related behaviors and their impact on daily functioning.

5. Cognitive and Neuropsychological Testing: These tests assess various cognitive functions, such as attention, memory, and executive functioning, providing a comprehensive evaluation of the individual's cognitive profile.

Working with Healthcare Professionals and Specialists: Collaboration with healthcare professionals and specialists is crucial throughout the evaluation process.
Here are some important considerations:

1. Seek a Qualified Healthcare Professional: It is important to work with a healthcare professional who specializes in ADHD and has experience in diagnosing and treating the disorder. Psychiatrists, psychologists, or pediatricians with expertise in ADHD are well-equipped to conduct a comprehensive evaluation.

2. Provide Comprehensive Information: Be prepared to provide a detailed account of the individual's symptoms, history, and any relevant information that may help in the evaluation process. This includes information from different settings, such as school reports or teacher observations.

3. Open and Honest Communication: Maintain open and honest communication with the healthcare professional, sharing any concerns, questions, or observations related to the individual's symptoms and behaviors. This collaborative approach helps ensure an accurate assessment and appropriate treatment planning.

4. Multidisciplinary Approach: In some cases, collaborating with other healthcare professionals, such as educational specialists or occupational therapists, can provide a comprehensive evaluation and inform the development of an individualized treatment plan.

Remember, an ADHD diagnosis should never be based on a single assessment or evaluation. A comprehensive evaluation process, involving multiple sources of information and professional expertise, ensures a more accurate diagnosis and enables the development of an effective treatment plan.

In conclusion, obtaining an ADHD diagnosis involves a comprehensive evaluation process conducted by qualified healthcare professionals. The assessment may include clinical interviews, rating scales, medical and developmental history reviews, behavioral observations, and cognitive testing. Collaborating with healthcare professionals and specialists is crucial for accurate diagnosis and the development of an individualized treatment plan. By following this collaborative approach, individuals with ADHD can receive the support and interventions they need to manage their symptoms and improve their quality of life.

Chapter 4: Understanding ADHD Treatment Options

When it comes to managing Attention-Deficit/Hyperactivity Disorder (ADHD), there are various treatment options available. This section will explore the three main approaches to ADHD treatment: medication, behavioral therapy, and alternative and complementary therapies. Each option has its own benefits, risks, and considerations, and a combination of approaches may be recommended based on individual needs.

Medication:

Medication is a common treatment approach for ADHD and can be effective in managing symptoms. Stimulant medications, such as methylphenidate and amphetamines, are often prescribed and work by increasing certain neurotransmitters in the brain that regulate attention and impulse control. Non-stimulant medications, such as atomoxetine, may be recommended for those who do not respond well to or have contraindications for stimulant medications.

Benefits: Medication can help improve attention, reduce impulsivity and hyperactivity, and enhance overall functioning. It can provide short-term symptom relief and may be particularly helpful in academic or work settings.

Risks and Considerations: Like any medication, ADHD medications have potential side effects, such as decreased appetite, difficulty sleeping, or increased heart rate. Close monitoring by a healthcare professional is necessary to ensure safety and efficacy. Additionally, medication is not a cure and should be used in conjunction with other treatment strategies.

Behavioral Therapy:
Behavioral therapy is a non-pharmacological approach that focuses on teaching individuals with ADHD specific strategies and techniques to manage their symptoms and improve functioning. This type of therapy is often used in combination with medication or as a stand-alone treatment.

Strategies and Techniques: Behavioral therapy for ADHD may include:

- **Psychoeducation**: Educating individuals and their families about ADHD, its symptoms, and management strategies.

- **Parent Training**: Providing parents with strategies to support their child's behavior, structure routines, and implement consistent discipline.
- **Cognitive-Behavioral Therapy (CBT)**: Teaching individuals to identify and challenge negative thought patterns, improve problem-solving skills, and develop coping strategies.
- **Social Skills Training**: Helping individuals improve their social interactions, communication skills, and conflict resolution abilities.

Behavioral therapy focuses on skill-building and can be tailored to address specific areas of difficulty for each individual.

Alternative and Complementary Therapies:

Alternative and complementary therapies encompass a wide range of approaches that are used alongside or as alternatives to conventional treatments. While the evidence supporting their effectiveness for ADHD is limited, some individuals find these therapies helpful in managing symptoms and improving overall well-being.
 Examples include:

- **Mindfulness and Meditation**: Practices that promote relaxation, self-awareness, and attention regulation.

- **Neurofeedback**: A form of biofeedback that aims to train individuals to self-regulate brainwave patterns associated with attention and focus.

- **Dietary and Nutritional Interventions**: Some individuals may explore dietary changes, such as eliminating certain food additives or increasing omega-3 fatty acids, to support brain health. However, evidence for their effectiveness is limited.

It's important to note that alternative and complementary therapies should be approached with caution and in consultation with healthcare professionals. They should not be used as a substitute for evidence-based treatments but rather as complementary additions.

In conclusion, ADHD treatment options include medication, behavioral therapy, and alternative and complementary therapies. Medication can provide short-term symptom relief, while behavioral therapy focuses on skill-building and strategies for managing symptoms. Alternative and complementary therapies may be explored as complementary additions, although evidence for their effectiveness is limited. A comprehensive treatment approach, tailored to individual needs, may involve a combination of these options. Consulting with healthcare professionals and specialists is essential to determine the most appropriate treatment plan for managing ADHD.

Chapter 5: Creating a Supportive Home Environment

A supportive home environment plays a crucial role in helping individuals with Attention-Deficit/Hyperactivity Disorder (ADHD) manage their symptoms and thrive. By implementing certain strategies and structures, families can provide the necessary support and create an environment conducive to success. This section will explore three key aspects of creating a supportive home environment: establishing routines and structure, effective communication strategies, and setting up a conducive study and homework area.

Establishing Routines and Structure:

Routines and structure provide predictability and help individuals with ADHD better manage their time and tasks. Consider the following:

- **Daily Schedule**: Establish a consistent daily routine with set times for waking up, meals, homework, and bedtime. Display the schedule visibly to serve as a reminder.

- Clear Expectations: Clearly communicate expectations regarding responsibilities and behavior. Break tasks into manageable steps and provide visual cues or checklists to assist with organization.

- Consistent Rules and Consequences: Establish consistent rules and consequences for behavior. Clearly communicate these rules and reinforce positive behaviors through praise and rewards.

Effective Communication Strategies:
Communication plays a crucial role in understanding and supporting individuals with ADHD. Consider the following strategies:

- Active Listening: Practice active listening by giving full attention, maintaining eye contact, and providing verbal and non-verbal cues to show understanding.

- Clear and Concise Instructions: Use simple, clear, and concise instructions to help individuals with ADHD understand and follow directions. Break tasks into smaller, manageable steps.

- **Use Visual Supports**: Visual aids, such as charts, calendars, or reminder boards, can be helpful in conveying information and reinforcing expectations.

- **Positive Reinforcement**: Offer praise and positive reinforcement when individuals with ADHD demonstrate desired behaviors or accomplish tasks.

Setting up a Conducive Study and Homework Area: Creating an organized and distraction-free study area can greatly benefit individuals with ADHD. Consider the following tips:

- **Reduce Distractions**: Minimize distractions in the study area by eliminating or reducing visual and auditory stimuli. Consider using noise-canceling headphones or white noise machines.

- **Organize Materials**: Provide storage solutions, such as labeled bins or folders, to help individuals with ADHD keep their study materials organized and easily accessible.

- **Clear Workspace**: Ensure the study area has ample space for materials and work surfaces. Remove unnecessary clutter and distractions.

- **Time Management Tools**: Use visual timers or apps to help individuals with ADHD manage their time effectively and stay on task.

- **Breaks and Movement**: Encourage short breaks during study sessions to allow for movement and reduce restlessness. Incorporate physical activity or movement breaks to help maintain focus.

By implementing these strategies and creating a supportive home environment, families can provide structure, clear communication, and a conducive space for individuals with ADHD to thrive. It is important to tailor these approaches to the specific needs and preferences of the individual, while also encouraging their active participation in developing strategies that work best for them.

Chapter 6: Managing ADHD at School

Managing Attention-Deficit/Hyperactivity Disorder (ADHD) at school requires effective collaboration between parents, teachers, and school staff. By working together and implementing strategies to support the needs of students with ADHD, a positive and inclusive learning environment can be fostered. This section will discuss three key aspects of managing ADHD at school: collaborating with teachers and school staff, developing individualized education plans (IEPs), and advocating for your child's needs.

Collaborating with Teachers and School Staff:
Open and ongoing communication between parents and teachers is crucial for supporting students with ADHD. Consider the following strategies:

- **Share Information**: Provide teachers with relevant information about your child's ADHD diagnosis, symptoms, and any recommended accommodations or strategies.

- **Establish Regular Communication**: Schedule regular check-ins or meetings with teachers to discuss your child's progress, challenges, and strategies that have been effective.

- **Share Successful Strategies**: Inform teachers about strategies that work well for your child, such as visual aids, preferential seating, or frequent check-ins to ensure understanding and engagement.

- **Consistency and Coordination**: Collaborate with teachers to ensure consistency in expectations, routines, and consequences between home and school. This helps create a structured and predictable environment for the student.

Developing Individualized Education Plans (IEPs):
An Individualized Education Plan (IEP) is a legally binding document that outlines specific accommodations, modifications, and support services for students with disabilities, including ADHD. Consider the following steps:

- **Request an IEP Meeting**: Initiate a meeting with the school's special education team to discuss the need for an IEP for your child. Present relevant documentation, such as medical reports or assessments, to support the request.

- **Participate in the IEP Process**: Attend the IEP meeting and actively contribute to the development of the plan. Share your insights, concerns, and goals for your child's education. Collaborate with the team to identify appropriate accommodations and supports.

- **Define Accommodations and Supports**: Work with the IEP team to establish accommodations and modifications that address your child's specific needs, such as extended time on assignments, preferential seating, or the use of assistive technology.

- **Regular Review and Updates**: Review the IEP regularly with the school team to ensure its effectiveness and make any necessary adjustments. Provide feedback and share updates on your child's progress and challenges.

Advocating for Your Child's Needs:
Advocacy plays a crucial role in ensuring that your child's educational needs are met. Consider the following strategies:

- **Educate Yourself**: Learn about your child's rights and entitlements under the Individuals with Disabilities Education Act (IDEA) or similar legislation in your region.

Understand the resources and support available to students with ADHD.

- **Assertive Communication**: Be proactive and assertive in communicating your child's needs to school staff. Clearly express your concerns and expectations, and seek clarification on any areas that require further explanation.

- **Request Accommodations**: If you believe additional accommodations or supports are needed, formally request a meeting with the school to discuss your concerns. Present supporting evidence, such as professional evaluations or recommendations.

- **Build a Support Network**: Connect with other parents of children with ADHD to share experiences, advice, and resources. Join support groups or advocacy organizations that can provide guidance and support.

Remember, effective management of ADHD at school requires ongoing collaboration, open communication, and advocating for your child's needs. By working together with teachers and school staff, developing an IEP, and advocating for appropriate accommodations, you can create a supportive and inclusive learning environment that maximizes your child's potential.

Chapter 7: Enhancing Social Skills and Peer Relationships

Developing strong social skills and fostering positive peer relationships are vital for individuals with Attention-Deficit/Hyperactivity Disorder (ADHD) to thrive socially and emotionally. By nurturing friendships, addressing bullying and teasing, and promoting self-esteem and self-advocacy, individuals with ADHD can build meaningful connections and navigate social interactions more effectively. This section will explore three key aspects of enhancing social skills and peer relationships for individuals with ADHD.

Nurturing Friendships and Social Interactions:
Encouraging and supporting the development of friendships and positive social interactions can greatly benefit individuals with ADHD. Consider the following strategies:

- **Teach Social Skills**: Provide explicit instruction on social skills, such as active listening, initiating conversations, sharing, taking turns, and resolving conflicts. Role-playing and social stories can be helpful tools.

- Encourage Extracurricular Activities: Encourage participation in extracurricular activities or clubs that align with your child's interests. These provide opportunities to meet peers with similar interests and build social connections.

- Facilitate Social Opportunities: Arrange playdates or outings with classmates or friends outside of school to provide more relaxed and controlled environments for social interaction.

- Promote Empathy and Perspective-Taking: Help individuals with ADHD develop empathy by encouraging them to consider others' feelings and perspectives. Teach them to be mindful of social cues and non-verbal communication.

Dealing with Bullying and Teasing:
Bullying and teasing can be particularly challenging for individuals with ADHD. It is important to address and respond to these situations appropriately. Consider the following strategies:

- **Open Communication**: Foster open communication with your child, encouraging them to share their experiences and emotions. Create a safe space where they feel comfortable discussing any incidents of bullying or teasing.

- **Teach Assertiveness Skills**: Help your child develop assertiveness skills to respond to bullying situations appropriately. This includes teaching them to use "I" statements, express their feelings calmly, and seek help from trusted adults.

- **Work with School Staff**: Inform teachers and school staff about any incidents of bullying or teasing, ensuring they are aware of the situation and can intervene appropriately. Collaborate with the school to develop strategies to address and prevent bullying.

- **Build Resilience**: Help your child develop resilience and coping strategies to deal with bullying. Encourage them to focus on their strengths, surround themselves with supportive friends, and seek help from trusted adults.

Promoting Self-Esteem and Self-Advocacy:

Promoting self-esteem and self-advocacy empowers individuals with ADHD to assert their needs and navigate social situations more effectively.

Consider the following strategies:

- **Recognize Strengths**: Highlight and celebrate your child's strengths and accomplishments. Encourage them to recognize their unique qualities and contributions.

- **Encourage Self-Expression**: Support your child's self-expression through creative outlets such as art, music, or writing. This can help boost self-esteem and provide a sense of accomplishment.

- **Teach Self-Advocacy Skills**: Help your child develop self-advocacy skills, such as expressing their needs, asking for help when necessary, and seeking accommodations or support from teachers and other trusted adults.

- **Provide Supportive Feedback**: Offer constructive and supportive feedback to help your child develop a positive self-image and encourage them to take pride in their efforts and progress.

By nurturing friendships, addressing bullying, and promoting self-esteem and self-advocacy, individuals with ADHD can develop the social skills and confidence needed to navigate social situations successfully. It is important to provide ongoing support, open communication, and reinforcement of positive behaviors to help individuals with ADHD thrive socially and build meaningful connections with their peers.

Chapter 8: Coping with ADHD-Related Challenges

Individuals with Attention-Deficit/Hyperactivity Disorder (ADHD) often face specific challenges related to time management, organization, impulsivity, self-control, and emotional regulation. By implementing effective coping strategies, individuals with ADHD can better navigate these challenges and improve their overall functioning. This section will explore three key areas of coping with ADHD-related challenges: time management and organization skills, impulsivity and self-control strategies, and dealing with emotional regulation difficulties.

Time Management and Organization Skills:
Managing time and staying organized can be particularly challenging for individuals with ADHD. Here are some strategies to cope with these difficulties:

- **Use Visual Aids**: Utilize visual tools such as calendars, to-do lists, and reminders to help organize tasks and appointments. Display them prominently in visible locations.

- **Break Tasks into Smaller Steps**: Large tasks can feel overwhelming. Break them down into smaller, more manageable steps to make them less daunting and easier to approach.

- **Prioritize Tasks**: Teach individuals with ADHD to prioritize tasks based on importance and deadline. Encourage them to tackle high-priority tasks first and use time-blocking techniques to allocate specific time slots for different activities.

- **Set Timers and Alarms**: Use timers or alarms to help individuals with ADHD stay on track and manage time effectively. This can be especially useful for transitioning between tasks or completing assignments within a specified timeframe.

Impulsivity and Self-Control Strategies:
Impulsivity and difficulties with self-control are common challenges for individuals with ADHD. The following strategies can help manage impulsive behaviors and enhance self-control:

- **Take a Pause**: Encourage individuals with ADHD to pause and take a deep breath before acting on impulsive urges. Taking a moment to reflect can help interrupt impulsive behavior.

- **Use "Stop and Think" Strategies**: Teach individuals to use "stop and think" techniques, such as mentally counting to ten or considering the potential consequences before responding or acting impulsively.

- **Practice Delayed Gratification**: Encourage individuals to practice delayed gratification by setting goals and rewarding themselves after completing tasks or achieving milestones. This helps develop patience and self-control.

- **Implement Self-Monitoring**: Foster self-awareness by helping individuals recognize their impulsive behaviors. Encourage self-monitoring techniques, such as keeping a journal or using apps that track impulsive tendencies, to promote self-reflection and awareness.

Dealing with Emotional Regulation Difficulties:
Emotional regulation can be challenging for individuals with ADHD. The following strategies can help manage and regulate emotions effectively:

- **Develop Emotional Awareness**: Help individuals with ADHD recognize and label their emotions. Encourage them to identify their emotional triggers and patterns, which can aid in developing appropriate coping strategies.

- **Practice Relaxation Techniques**: Teach relaxation techniques, such as deep breathing exercises, mindfulness, or progressive muscle relaxation, to help manage emotional intensity and promote a sense of calm.

- **Encourage Healthy Coping Mechanisms**: Promote healthy ways of coping with emotions, such as engaging in physical exercise, pursuing hobbies, writing in a journal, or talking to a trusted friend or family member.

- **Seek Support**: Encourage individuals to seek support from therapists, counselors, or support groups to learn additional coping skills and strategies for managing emotions effectively.

By implementing these coping strategies, individuals with ADHD can develop essential skills to manage time, control impulsive behaviors, and regulate emotions. It's important to provide ongoing support, patience, and reinforcement of positive efforts as individuals work on coping with ADHD-related challenges.

Chapter 9: Supporting Positive Behavior and Discipline

Supporting positive behavior and implementing effective discipline strategies are important for individuals with Attention-Deficit/Hyperactivity Disorder (ADHD) to thrive and develop appropriate self-regulation skills. By using techniques that promote positive behavior, finding the right balance between rewards and consequences, and encouraging self-monitoring and self-regulation, individuals with ADHD can enhance their overall behavior and well-being. This section will explore three key aspects of supporting positive behavior and discipline for individuals with ADHD.

Implementing Effective Behavior Management Techniques:

Effective behavior management techniques can help individuals with ADHD develop and maintain positive behavior. Consider the following strategies:

- **Clear Expectations**: Clearly communicate expectations and rules to individuals with ADHD. Use concise and specific language to help them understand what is expected of them in different situations.

- **Positive Reinforcement**: Implement a system of rewards and praise to reinforce positive behaviors. Recognize and acknowledge efforts and achievements, whether big or small. This encourages motivation and reinforces desired behavior.

- **Consistency and Predictability**: Establish consistent routines and predictable environments. Individuals with ADHD thrive in structured environments, where they know what to expect. Consistency helps reduce anxiety and supports the development of positive behavior patterns.

- **Use Visual Supports**: Utilize visual aids, such as behavior charts or token systems, to help individuals track and monitor their behavior. Visual supports provide clear feedback and allow for self-reflection.

Rewards and Consequences: Finding the Right Balance:

Finding the right balance between rewards and consequences is essential in supporting positive behavior and discipline for individuals with ADHD. Consider the following strategies:

- Emphasize Positive Reinforcement: Place a strong emphasis on positive reinforcement to motivate and encourage desired behaviors. This includes verbal praise, tangible rewards, or privileges.

- Use Consequences Effectively: Consequences should be clear, consistent, and proportionate to the behavior. Focus on natural consequences, whenever possible, to help individuals learn from their actions. Ensure consequences are implemented in a calm and non-punitive manner.

- Encourage Reflection: Instead of solely relying on external consequences, encourage individuals to reflect on their behavior and its impact on themselves and others. This helps develop internal motivation and self-awareness.

- Individualize Strategies: Each individual with ADHD is unique, so it's important to tailor rewards and consequences to their specific needs and preferences. Experiment with different approaches to find what works best for them.

Promoting Self-Monitoring and Self-Regulation: Promoting self-monitoring and self-regulation skills empowers individuals with ADHD to become active participants in managing their behavior. Consider the following strategies:

- **Teach Self-Awareness**: Help individuals with ADHD develop self-awareness by encouraging them to recognize their thoughts, emotions, and behavior patterns. This allows them to identify triggers and make conscious choices.

- **Goal Setting**: Support individuals in setting realistic and achievable goals related to behavior and self-regulation. Break down larger goals into smaller, attainable steps, and celebrate progress along the way.

- **Self-Reflection and Problem-Solving**: Encourage individuals to engage in self-reflection and problem-solving. This involves identifying challenges, brainstorming alternative solutions, and evaluating the effectiveness of their choices.

- **Provide Tools for Self-Regulation**: Teach individuals coping strategies and self-regulation techniques, such as deep breathing exercises, self-talk, or mindfulness, to help manage emotions and impulsive behaviors.

By implementing effective behavior management techniques, finding the right balance between rewards and consequences, and promoting self-monitoring and self-regulation, individuals with ADHD can develop positive behavior patterns and enhance their self-control and self-discipline. It is important to provide ongoing support, guidance, and reinforcement of positive efforts as individuals work on developing and maintaining positive behaviors.

Chapter 10: Addressing Coexisting Conditions and Challenges

Individuals with Attention-Deficit/Hyperactivity Disorder (ADHD) often experience coexisting conditions or face additional challenges that can impact their well-being and daily functioning. Addressing these coexisting conditions and challenges is essential for providing comprehensive support. This section will explore three common coexisting conditions and challenges: anxiety and depression, learning disabilities, and sleep problems, in relation to ADHD.

Anxiety, Depression, and ADHD:
Anxiety and depression frequently coexist with ADHD, as individuals with ADHD may experience challenges related to attention, impulsivity, and social interactions. Here are some considerations:

- **Recognize Symptoms**: Be aware of signs and symptoms of anxiety and depression, such as excessive worry, low mood, withdrawal, or changes in sleep and appetite. Consult with healthcare professionals to assess and address these conditions.

- **Treatment Approaches**: Treatment for anxiety and depression may include therapy, medication, or a combination of both. Cognitive-Behavioral Therapy (CBT) can be particularly helpful in addressing anxiety and depression in individuals with ADHD.

- **Collaborate with Professionals**: Work with healthcare professionals, therapists, and educators to develop strategies that support both ADHD management and the treatment of anxiety and depression. This collaborative approach ensures comprehensive care and support.

Learning Disabilities and ADHD:
ADHD often coexists with learning disabilities, such as dyslexia, dyscalculia, or specific language impairments. Addressing these challenges requires a tailored approach:

- **Identify Learning Disabilities**: If you suspect a learning disability, consult with educators, school psychologists, or other specialists to conduct a comprehensive evaluation. This helps determine specific learning challenges and develop appropriate interventions.

- **Individualized Education Plan (IEP)**: Collaborate with the school to develop an IEP that addresses both ADHD and learning disabilities. Ensure accommodations, modifications, and specialized instruction are provided to support academic progress.

- **Supportive Interventions**: Implement strategies that support learning, such as providing assistive technology, using multisensory approaches, or offering additional academic support. Utilize individualized instruction and provide opportunities for repetition and reinforcement.

Sleep Problems and ADHD:
Individuals with ADHD often experience sleep problems, including difficulties with falling asleep, staying asleep, or maintaining a regular sleep schedule. Addressing these issues can improve overall well-being:

- **Establish Bedtime Routine**: Develop a consistent and calming bedtime routine to signal the body and mind that it is time to wind down. Encourage activities such as reading, relaxation exercises, or listening to soothing music.

- **Promote Sleep Hygiene**: Encourage good sleep hygiene practices, such as keeping a regular sleep schedule, creating a sleep-friendly environment (e.g., reducing noise and light), and avoiding stimulating activities close to bedtime.

- Consult with Healthcare Professionals: If sleep problems persist, consult with healthcare professionals to assess and address any underlying issues. They may recommend behavioral interventions, medication (if necessary), or other strategies to improve sleep quality.

It is crucial to seek professional guidance and support when addressing coexisting conditions and challenges related to ADHD. Collaborating with healthcare professionals, educators, and specialists ensures a comprehensive approach to managing ADHD and addressing the specific needs associated with coexisting conditions. By addressing these challenges, individuals with ADHD can receive the necessary support to enhance their overall well-being and quality of life.

Chapter 11: Nurturing Strengths and Building Resilience

Nurturing strengths and building resilience are essential for individuals with Attention-Deficit/Hyperactivity Disorder (ADHD) to develop a positive self-image, embrace their unique talents, and overcome challenges. By identifying and cultivating individual talents, encouraging self-advocacy and self-awareness, and fostering a growth mindset, individuals with ADHD can build resilience and thrive. This section will explore three key aspects of nurturing strengths and building resilience for individuals with ADHD.

Identifying and Cultivating Individual Talents:
Recognizing and cultivating individual talents can help individuals with ADHD develop a sense of purpose and accomplishment. Consider the following strategies:

- **Encourage Exploration**: Provide opportunities for individuals with ADHD to explore different interests, hobbies, and activities. Allow them to discover their passions and strengths.

- **Offer Supportive Environments**: Create an environment that values and celebrates individual talents. Provide resources, materials, or classes that align with their interests and talents.

- **Focus on Strengths**: Shift the focus from weaknesses to strengths. Help individuals identify their unique strengths, such as creativity, problem-solving abilities, or out-of-the-box thinking. Encourage them to utilize these strengths in various aspects of their lives.

Encouraging Self-Advocacy and Self-Awareness:
Promoting self-advocacy and self-awareness empowers individuals with ADHD to understand their needs, advocate for themselves, and navigate challenges effectively. Consider the following strategies:

- **Teach Self-Advocacy Skills**: Help individuals with ADHD understand their rights and educate them about their specific needs related to ADHD. Encourage them to communicate their needs to teachers, peers, and other relevant individuals.

- **Foster Self-Awareness**: Promote self-reflection and self-awareness by encouraging individuals to recognize their strengths, challenges, and emotions. Help them develop a better understanding of their own behavior, triggers, and coping strategies.

- Provide Tools for Self-Expression: Teach individuals effective communication skills, including active listening, expressing emotions assertively, and problem-solving. These skills facilitate self-advocacy and help build positive relationships.

Fostering a Growth Mindset:
Developing a growth mindset can enhance resilience and foster a positive attitude toward challenges and setbacks. Consider the following strategies:

- Embrace Mistakes as Opportunities: Encourage individuals to view mistakes as opportunities for growth and learning. Help them understand that setbacks are a natural part of the learning process and can lead to improvement.

- Promote Effort and Persistence: Emphasize the value of effort and perseverance over immediate success. Encourage individuals to embrace challenges, put in the necessary effort, and persist even when faced with difficulties.

- **Provide Encouragement and Support**: Offer praise and encouragement for effort, progress, and the development of new skills. Provide support during challenging times and remind individuals of their ability to overcome obstacles.

- **Set Realistic Goals**: Help individuals set realistic and achievable goals that stretch their abilities. Break larger goals into smaller, manageable steps to provide a sense of accomplishment along the way.

By nurturing strengths, encouraging self-advocacy and self-awareness, and fostering a growth mindset, individuals with ADHD can build resilience and develop a positive self-image. It is important to provide ongoing support, guidance, and reinforcement of their efforts. With these strategies, individuals with ADHD can thrive and reach their full potential.

Chapter 12: Taking Care of Yourself: Parent and Caregiver Well-being

Caring for a child with Attention-Deficit/Hyperactivity Disorder (ADHD) can be demanding and challenging, making it essential for parents and caregivers to prioritize their own well-being. By managing stress and burnout, seeking support and building a network, and prioritizing self-care and personal needs, parents and caregivers can maintain their own health and well-being. This section will explore three key aspects of taking care of yourself as a parent or caregiver of a child with ADHD.

Managing Stress and Burnout:

Managing stress and preventing burnout is crucial for maintaining your own well-being while caring for a child with ADHD. Consider the following strategies:

- **Establish Boundaries**: Set clear boundaries between your caregiving responsibilities and personal time. Learn to say no when necessary and prioritize activities that help you relax and recharge.

- **Practice Stress-Management Techniques**: Incorporate stress-reducing activities into your routine, such as exercise, meditation, deep breathing exercises, or engaging in hobbies. Find what works best for you to alleviate stress and promote relaxation.

- **Time Management**: Develop effective time-management strategies to balance your caregiving responsibilities with other aspects of your life. Prioritize tasks, delegate when possible, and identify time for self-care and personal activities.

Seeking Support and Building a Network:
Seeking support and building a network of understanding individuals can provide a valuable source of encouragement and resources. Consider the following strategies:

- **Join Support Groups**: Connect with other parents and caregivers who are also caring for children with ADHD. Sharing experiences, insights, and advice can provide a sense of community and support.

- **Seek Professional Support**: Consider reaching out to therapists, counselors, or support groups specifically tailored to parents and caregivers of children with ADHD.

Professional guidance can provide valuable strategies for coping with challenges and enhancing your well-being.

- Communicate with Family and Friends: Keep the lines of communication open with family and friends. Share your experiences, concerns, and needs, and let them know how they can support you.

Prioritizing Self-Care and Personal Needs:
Prioritizing self-care and attending to your own needs is essential for maintaining your physical and emotional well-being. Consider the following strategies:

- Self-Care Routine: Establish a regular self-care routine that includes activities you enjoy and that help you relax and recharge. This can include activities such as exercise, reading, spending time in nature, practicing mindfulness, or pursuing hobbies.

- Delegate and Accept Help: Recognize that it is okay to ask for and accept help. Delegate tasks to other family members or trusted individuals, and be open to accepting support when it is offered.

- Practice Self-Compassion: Be kind and compassionate towards yourself. Acknowledge that you are doing your best, and give yourself permission to prioritize your well-being and personal needs.

- Take Breaks: Allow yourself breaks and moments of respite. Step away from caregiving responsibilities and engage in activities that bring you joy and relaxation. Taking care of yourself enables you to better support your child with ADHD.

Remember, taking care of yourself is not selfish but necessary for your own well-being and your ability to care for your child with ADHD. By managing stress and burnout, seeking support, and prioritizing self-care, you can maintain your own health and find the strength and resilience needed to navigate the challenges of parenting a child with ADHD.

Chapter 13: Transitioning to Adolescence and Adulthood

The transition from childhood to adolescence and adulthood can bring about unique challenges and changes for individuals with Attention-Deficit/Hyperactivity Disorder (ADHD). It is important to prepare for academic and vocational transitions, address the challenges associated with adolescence, and support the development of independence and self-management skills. This section will explore three key aspects of transitioning to adolescence and adulthood for individuals with ADHD.

Challenges and Changes during Adolescence:
Adolescence is a time of significant physical, emotional, and social changes. Individuals with ADHD may face specific challenges during this period. Consider the following strategies:

- **Education about Puberty**: Provide age-appropriate education about the physical and emotional changes of puberty. This helps individuals understand and cope with the changes they experience.

- **Emotional Support**: Offer emotional support and open communication channels to address the emotional challenges that can arise during adolescence. Encourage individuals to express their thoughts and feelings, and provide guidance on healthy coping strategies.

- **Developing Healthy Relationships**: Assist individuals in developing healthy peer relationships by teaching social skills, promoting empathy, and providing guidance on appropriate boundaries and conflict resolution.

Preparing for Academic and Vocational Transitions: Preparing for academic and vocational transitions is crucial as individuals with ADHD move toward adulthood. Consider the following strategies:

- **Individualized Transition Planning**: Collaborate with educators and specialists to develop individualized transition plans that address academic and vocational goals. Identify appropriate accommodations and supports to facilitate success during these transitions.

- **Career Exploration**: Encourage career exploration and provide opportunities for individuals to learn about various professions and interests. Offer guidance and support in aligning their passions and strengths with potential career paths.

- **Skill Development**: Help individuals develop essential skills for academic and vocational success, such as time management, organization, goal setting, and problem-solving. Support them in accessing resources and services that can assist in their skill development.

Building Independence and Self-Management Skills:
Building independence and self-management skills is critical for individuals with ADHD as they transition to adulthood. Consider the following strategies:

- **Gradual Responsibility**: Gradually increase responsibilities and allow individuals to practice independence in age-appropriate tasks. Provide support and guidance as needed, gradually stepping back to foster self-reliance.

- **Executive Functioning Strategies**: Teach and reinforce executive functioning strategies, such as planning, prioritizing, and breaking tasks into manageable steps. These skills enhance independence and self-management.

- **Self-Advocacy**: Encourage self-advocacy by helping individuals understand their rights, express their needs, and seek accommodations or support when necessary. Teach them how to effectively communicate with teachers, employers, and other relevant individuals.

- **Financial Management Skills**: Support the development of financial management skills by teaching budgeting, saving, and responsible spending. Provide opportunities for individuals to practice managing their finances and make informed financial decisions.

By addressing the challenges and changes of adolescence, preparing for academic and vocational transitions, and promoting independence and self-management skills, individuals with ADHD can navigate the transition to adulthood more effectively. It is important to provide ongoing support, guidance, and reinforcement as they develop the skills and resilience needed for success in adult life.

Chapter 14: Celebrating Success and Progress

Celebrating success and progress is an important aspect of raising a child with Attention-Deficit/Hyperactivity Disorder (ADHD). By recognizing achievements, setting realistic expectations, and embracing the journey of raising a child with ADHD, parents and caregivers can create a positive and supportive environment that nurtures growth and self-esteem. This section will explore three key aspects of celebrating success and progress in the context of ADHD.

Recognizing Achievements, Big and Small:
Recognizing and celebrating achievements, big and small, helps boost self-confidence and reinforces positive behaviors. Consider the following strategies:

- **Celebrate Effort**: Acknowledge the effort your child puts into their tasks and activities. Recognize their determination and persistence, regardless of the outcome. Praise their commitment and hard work.

- **Highlight Progress**: Focus on the progress your child has made, rather than solely on the end result. Recognize improvements, whether they are academic, social, or personal. Emphasize growth and development over perfection.

- **Personalize Celebrations**: Tailor celebrations to your child's interests and preferences. Celebrate achievements in ways that are meaningful to them, such as planning a special outing, creating a personalized reward system, or having a family celebration.

Setting Realistic Expectations:

Setting realistic expectations is important for both the child and the parent or caregiver. It helps reduce stress and fosters a sense of accomplishment. Consider the following strategies:

- **Understand Individual Abilities**: Recognize and appreciate your child's unique strengths, challenges, and developmental stage. Set expectations that align with their abilities, considering their ADHD-related difficulties and any coexisting conditions.

- **Break Tasks into Smaller Steps**: Break down larger tasks or goals into smaller, manageable steps. This makes them more attainable and allows for a sense of progress and accomplishment along the way.

- **Focus on Personal Growth**: Encourage personal growth and improvement rather than comparing your child to others. Emphasize their individual journey and support them in reaching their full potential.

Embracing the Journey of Raising a Child with ADHD:

Embracing the journey of raising a child with ADHD involves accepting challenges, finding joy in small victories, and maintaining a positive outlook. Consider the following strategies:

- **Cultivate a Positive Mindset**: Focus on the strengths and positive qualities of your child. Cultivate a mindset that seeks solutions and growth opportunities rather than dwelling on limitations or setbacks.

- **Practice Self-Reflection**: Reflect on your own journey as a parent or caregiver. Recognize and celebrate your own progress, patience, and resilience. Acknowledge the dedication and love you bring to supporting your child.

- **Seek Support**: Connect with other parents or caregivers who are also raising children with ADHD. Share experiences, challenges, and successes. Support and learn from each other, finding comfort in knowing that you are not alone on this journey.

- **Celebrate Self-Care**: Take time to care for yourself, recharge, and seek support when needed. Remember that your well-being is essential for providing the support your child needs.

By recognizing achievements, setting realistic expectations, and embracing the journey of raising a child with ADHD, parents and caregivers can create an environment that fosters growth, resilience, and self-esteem. Celebrating success and progress not only benefits the child, but also acknowledges the efforts and dedication of the entire support system.

Conclusion

In conclusion, coping with Attention-Deficit/Hyperactivity Disorder (ADHD) as a parent or caregiver requires patience, understanding, and a comprehensive approach. Throughout this guide, we have explored various aspects of ADHD, from understanding its basics to addressing specific challenges and transitions. By implementing the strategies and recommendations provided, you can create a supportive and nurturing environment that fosters the well-being and development of individuals with ADHD.

We began by defining ADHD and dispelling myths and misconceptions surrounding it. We discussed the importance of recognizing symptoms, seeking a proper diagnosis, and understanding the prevalence of ADHD. From there, we delved into recognizing ADHD in children, understanding co-occurring conditions, and managing ADHD-related challenges. We also explored treatment options, creating a supportive home environment, managing ADHD at school, and enhancing social skills and peer relationships.

Taking care of yourself as a parent or caregiver is essential, and we discussed the importance of managing stress, seeking support, and prioritizing self-care. We also touched on the transitions to adolescence and adulthood, emphasizing the need for preparing individuals with ADHD for academic, vocational, and personal changes.

Throughout this journey, it is crucial to celebrate success and progress, setting realistic expectations and embracing the unique strengths of individuals with ADHD. By nurturing their talents, promoting self-advocacy, and fostering a growth mindset, we can help them build resilience and develop a positive self-image.

Remember, coping with ADHD is an ongoing process that requires adaptability and continuous learning. Each individual with ADHD is unique, and it is important to tailor strategies to their specific needs and strengths. By providing love, support, and understanding, you can empower individuals with ADHD to overcome challenges and thrive in their lives.

As a parent or caregiver, you are an invaluable source of guidance and support. Your commitment and dedication to the well-being of individuals with ADHD will make a significant impact on their lives. Together, we can create a nurturing environment where individuals with ADHD can reach their full potential and lead fulfilling and successful lives.